# THE BEAUTY PROFESSIONALS PLAYBOOK
## A Guide for New Beauty Professionals

## BY AMBER ROWE

# DEDICATION

This book is dedicated to my loving husband Isaac. If
not for your daily encouragement, support and
diligence none of this would be possible! .

# CONTENTS

# ACKNOWLEDGMENTS

I would like to acknowledge my family whose unconditional love and unwavering support has helped me through out my entire life. I also want to acknowledge my cosmetology instructors and mentors who believed in me and pushed me to be even greater than they were.

# INTRODUCTION

Do you have a passion for making others beautiful? Do you derive pleasure from fixing your friend or sister's hair? How often do you fix your nails and apply makeup? Do you have the habit of giving people beauty tips because you are naturally endowed with it?

If you are fond of any of these, then you have a passion for beauty. It won't be out of place then, to consider a career in the beauty industry.

Imagine being paid for what you naturally love doing? This is a once-in-a-lifetime opportunity to turn your passion into money-making machine. If you pursue your passion, you will experience contentment and fulfillment in life.

Perhaps you have some reservations. "How will I cope among so many students in the school?" "The industry is already saturated, what are the chances that I will be successful?" Are these your thoughts? Don't let these thoughts discourage you.

Remember the saying: "Do something that you love, and you will never have to work a day in your life."

How will you feel getting paid for something you'll naturally do for free?

To prepare you for a successful life in the beauty industry, I have written this book to serve as a guide to help you know what you need to do to make a success out of your hobby and passion. In this book, you will learn:

- Why you should consider a career in the beauty industry
- The job opportunities that are available for you
- How to pick the best school
- How you can build your unique brand
- How to retain customers, and much more.

Each of the points is discussed extensively to give you vital information that will help you overcome your apprehension, launch and promote your career and set it on a pedestal that will be the envy of all. I have invested 17 years into this industry and I can say that it's given me the ride of a lifetime! Early in my career I started out as a cosmetologist and I actually hated it. I'm glad that I figured it out early because there is nothing worse than doing something you DON'T love. Like most of you I got into the beauty industry because I loved beautiful hair, nails and makeup.

When I was in beauty school I invited all my friends over for haircuts. Some styles were better than others and I made quite a few mistakes! Over all, when you become a stylist or barber everyone wants to be your friend because you can offer them a better version of themselves. You have the potential to give your clients more confidence and self esteem. I wanted to write this book for new beauty professionals because if I had a mentor in the beginning of my career I wouldn't have had as many bumps along the road. I've been scammed by a beauty school, dealt with gossiping beauty professionals and had been treated unfairly by clients. I didn't know how to navigate all these things emotionally, physically or spiritually. My passion is to help you prepare for one of the best decisions you will make in your life. Choosing the beauty or wellness industry is a big deal. If you have this book in your hand you are thinking about what area of beauty you're interested in or you're out of beauty school and you're waiting to take your state exams. You may be waiting for your test results or on your second try at the exam. Maybe you're a new manicurist, massage therapist or hairstylist building new clientele. No matter where you are in the process, what you do now will affect the future of your career. So are you ready?

# CHAPTER 1

## MY PATH

My journey began while I was in high school, I had taken some courses at the local community college and I was bored out of my mind. I wanted to do what was traditional you know, the career plan your counselors talked about in school. And I did it because I really didn't know what I wanted to do with my career. I didn't want to take a summer off because I wasn't motivated enough to go back to classes. The military was an option but it just wasn't for me but I saw it as a last resort. So because of the stress I felt from my lack of direction, I decided to go to the spa with my sister! Upon arrival my sister and I were visually impressed with the overall look the spa. When we checked in at the front desk, my sister had her appointments on the books but I didn't have mine. So with a disappointed tone I asked, is anything else was available? The concierge replied, a foot treatment was available and I graciously said no because I am the most ticklish person on the entire planet! So I just waited for my sister to be done in the waiting area, which was very relaxing. Then I got complacent and I asked to take a tour. During the tour I felt like I was in another world! The aroma, the beautifully decorated treatment rooms and mandarin collared uniforms drew me in. While taking all this in my tour guide showed me her area where she worked. Her area was a foot treatment room, far better than some of the corner shops that are so easy to find. She had her own manicurist suite for her services, which made her modalities look very exclusive. I liked everything she described because in my eyes she offered a unique "experience" to her guests. I asked her where she went to school and she gave me the number to the school she went to. To my surprise it was owned by the spa we were in at that very moment! I set an appointment, started school and voila! Now, after 17 years invested into this career I often think back on my small beginnings. If it weren't for that young lady at the spa who took time out of her busy day to share valuable information with me, I don't know if I would have had to the courage to jump start my career. My career in the beauty industry has taken me from providing world-class spa treatments with exotic product lines to training and education for high-end spas nationally, seminars and workshops for beauty school students, freelance opportunities and independent contracts with businesses to improve customer service and efficiency. I've also worked on high fashion photo-shoots and also had a few house calls for a few celebrities. My experience in this industry has taught me more than skill set, it has taught me how to conduct myself in a professional manner. Learned how to work with people from all walks of life and how to be a servant leader, which we will talk about later. I am confident that this book will help you gain a new perspective on your new journey. You may be thinking - this pro nail technician is going to give me tips on my career path? Just bear with me and learn from my experiences. This opportunity if you choose to take it, doesn't have to just be a job, this can be whatever you want it to be. All you have to do is believe in yourself and decide that you will not give up, I didn't give up and it's taken me on the ride of a lifetime and I hope that even more comes to you! In the next chapter we will talk about why you may want to embark on this journey.

# CHAPTER 2

## TOP 5 REASONS WHY YOU SHOULD BE IN THE BEAUTY INDUSTRY

The beauty industry is now considered as one of the most flourishing industries in the world. For this reason, it is a gold mine for people who are naturally beauty-conscious or passionate to learn the culture of the industry. These are four of the main reasons why you should consider giving the industry a shot.

**Unlimited Creativity:**

The industry affords you the opportunity to express yourself. As a matter of fact, you can let your creativity do the talking while you focus on some other aspects of the industry that will contribute to your success. In view of the daily evolution in the fashion and beauty world, you can leverage on your creativity to stand out of the pack, beautifying people day in day out, and making money in the process.

**Job Flexibility:**

Instead of being stuck to a 9-to-5-work regimen, as a freelance hair stylist, you have absolute control over your time. You can take advantage of the flexibility of your job to engage yourself in other productive activities. What about the opportunity to attend awesome fashion shows and exciting photo shoots? These opportunities make a career in the beauty industry alluring and fun.

**Your Career Opportunities Are Limitless:**

Can you imagine the avalanche of job opportunities that are available to you as a professional beauty practitioner? You can work in spas, salon, and beauty school as an instructor or in any organization that has a stake in the fashion/beauty world. You are limited by your ability. If you are on top of your game, you have limitless career opportunities, and limitless opportunities to get paid for your services.

**It Is Easy To Build A Good Client Base:**

This is one of the major benefits of this profession. If you can combine your expertise with professionalism, you will take your passion to a higher level as your clients will "advertise" your services via words of mouth. And of course, you can't beat the power of word of mouth recommendation we'll talk about that later in the book.

**You Will Get Paid For Your Passion:**

Don't you consider it exciting to be paid for your passion? This will make the career easy and fun for you. You don't have to struggle to make ends meet while pursuing your passion and you won't have to sacrifice your passion for your career. Rather, you will be able to eat your cake and have it. That's fun, right? There is no denying that your passion and talent will take you to places. But, won't it be a better idea to hone your skills? If you enroll in a reputable beauty school, professionals who have been there and have known the prerequisites for success will be available to put finishing touches to your skills.

**There Comes Another Question:**

"Where should I enroll?" remember earlier in the book that was the first thing I asked my tour guide.

To bail you out of this predicament, I have developed some of the important qualities you must look for if you want to choose a beauty school to hone your skills. I have always shared this information with those considering the industry. My tips have results and still continue to guide potential beauty professionals in the right direction. In the next chapter I want to share more with you on how to pick the right educational platform for your future career.

# CHAPTER 3

## TOP QUALITIES OF A GOOD COSMETOLOGY SCHOOL

It must be accredited...Period

This is the first quality to look out for in a cosmetology school. An accredited school is under the auspices of the National Accrediting Commission for Career Arts & Sciences (NACCAS), as stipulated by the U.S. Department of Education. NACCASS has the objective of defining the curriculum and rules as well as set the standards that will ensure the efficiency and credibility of beauty school. Therefore, an accredited school is a good choice because it guarantees you good training and best industry practices and standards. Remember earlier I mentioned being scammed by a school that was accredited but under investigation. It's very important that you know the status of the school and if it has bad reviews before you invest your time and money. The general public can access this information by going online to your local commissions website or by calling your local state agencies. Remember each state is different but if you get online and key in words like, "cosmetology" and "state" your local agency should pop right up!

Apart from credibility, accreditation gives the students of such schools the eligibility to apply for financial aid from the government. This will surely lighten your financial responsibilities.

It must provide good professional training

Apart from teaching you the basic cosmetology skills, top cosmetology schools will give you extra training that will make you better equipped to handle the various job challenges that you may face in the future. This teaching may include how to adapt to changing tastes and styles in addition to making use of the latest and best resources in the field.

Business training should be included

There is more to being a beautician than fixing nails, styling hair, and what have you. You must know how to handle its slippery business terrain. A good beauty school will include professionalism training, ethics, and business management in its curriculum. Other important training should include resume building, how to handle a job interview, job-hunting, and how to impress potential clients. The training will arm you with the necessary business acumen to succeed in the beauty world so that you won't look out of place after your graduation.

Again, please consider graduation and dropout rates you can't afford not to consider this when scouting for a good cosmetology school. The higher the dropout rate, the lower the credibility of such school. On the other hand, if the graduation rates are high, that should instill some measure of confidence in you. For instance, if the dropout rates are high, find out what may be responsible for such a negative reputation. Again, the result of your findings may give you a clue into who the real problem is, the students or the school management. Regardless of the result of your investigation, you will have some basic information that will help you to make the right decision.

With these useful tips, you should be able to land yourself a top-notch cosmetology school where you will fine-tune your skills in preparation for a successful career in the beauty industry.

Now that you have gotten the beauty school of your dream, how can you make the best use of your time there? I know this is a lot of information but hang in there I've got you covered. Let me share the inside scoop with you I have 6 invaluable tips that'll help manage your time as a cosmetology student.

# CHAPTER 4

## 6 INVALUABLE TIPS THAT WILL MAKE YOU A SUCCESSFUL BEAUTY SCHOOL STUDENT

It takes diligence and dedication to become successful in any endeavor. To be successful as a beauty school student, cultivate these important qualities:

- **Punctuality:** People believe that "punctuality is the soul of business". Well, I will say it is not the soul of business alone; it is the soul of any successful endeavour. As a student, you should make it a habit to always show up for school and turn in your assignments before the deadlines. This will prepare you for the future of your career. Do you dream of being the best barber in the world? It is achievable if you work towards it. Don't forget that you can't be the best cosmetologist if you turn in late for school and graduate at the bottom of the class.

Therefore, the first step you need to take to get the best out of your beauty school is to embrace punctuality.

- **Be well dressed:** Your dressing and grooming speak volumes of your personality. If you can complement your punctuality with a wardrobe that oozes out class, you will feel confident among your colleagues and instructors. You will be the envy of all rather than being an object of ridicule. That will create an environment that is conducive to learning for you. If you can carry this trait over to your business after school, you will go places.

- **Make friends:** Well, you can't be the only new student in your school; there are other students who are new and feel out of place too. Mix with some of these new students to fight off loneliness. Over time, you can leverage your friendship to reflect positively on your academic performance. How? You can form a study group with fellow students and use the group to widen your academic horizon and knowledge. Treat topics together and make suggestions that will improve your rate of assimilation.

- **Ask questions:** You may find this suggestion very difficult to practice out of fear of being jeered by your colleague. Come to think of it, why did you enroll in the school? To learn, right? Would you have enrolled if you knew everything about the profession? Instead of focusing on the possible reactions of your peers, focus on the bigger picture: being a successful beauty student now and the best in the business in the future. Let that motivate you to overcome any potential element of discouragement in your quest to acquire the right skills to have a brilliant career and future. Ask reasonable questions and you will become knowledgeable.

- **Ask for help:** No matter you level of education we all have different ways of learning. Some of us are visual learners we watch something once and we got it. While others read and research, quite a few of us are audible. We hear instructions and do it perfectly to a tee. No matter how you learn be patient with yourself.

Whether English is your second language, math is a challenge or reading and writing. Most schools do require a GED or High school diploma but if you have a few other challenges please ask for help your instructors want you to succeed but they can't help if they don't know.

- **Be diligent:** Diligence will play a role in you graduating from the school with your head held high. If you dutifully and diligently carry out your responsibilities without succumbing to the pressure to handle your education flippantly, your grades will improve and your overall knowledge will be enough to see you through school.

- 

**Replay**

- **Be on time**
- **Look your best**
- **Be respectful**
- **Complete your assignments**
- **Always position yourself to learn more**
- **Practice Practice Practice**

After your graduation comes the real challenge of how to distinguish yourself from the rest? What can you do to be recognized among the thousands of both new and well-established names in the industry? I'll talk about that next...

# CHAPTER 5

## WHAT'S NEXT?

Once you graduate you will be on top of the world and you should be you are a finisher and you crossed the finish line but you need a quick reality check! Sorry to burst your bubble but if you were the star in school that's nice but know that in the industry your star status will be non-existent. It's very a competitive field and those clients who paid 25 to 45 dollars for a service in beauty school are not the same clients that will pay 65 to 85 the bar is set higher now as should your skills. But if you get your mind right now you can save yourself some unnecessary frustration in the long run. So you're looking around the room at graduation and everyone seems to have it together right. Some ladies or gents are already connected with the top salon or spa in town. Some may have work lined up in makeup or nails. Others have dreams of runway work in New York and one even said they were going to start a salon. Sounds lofty right, and here you are just wanted to pay that 17K student loan. Well don't become nervous just think about what YOUR dreams and goals are and start evolving. Who are you? What do you stand for? How do you want people to see you and receive you? This all makes up your brand. Don't let anyone taint who you are or what you want out of life or your career. Personally I'm very Zen and Fierce because I love pedicures, essential oils and yoga pants. On the other hand I like makeup and high heels for when I'm on a fabulous fashion shoot! People would call me the YODA of the spa where I worked because I'm very peaceful and gave good advice. Sometimes after work I would rush off to invite only concerts with a backstage pass with full face of makeup and hair styled to freelance for a few celebrities! I love both spectrums so I had to learn how to be myself but also adapt. In some cases for instance, if you have tattoos but you want to work styling kids hair just wear a long-sleeve shirt! If you are a wild child with purple hair and your employer wants you to have less vibrant colors in your hair are you willing to adjust because its is your dream job? How about applying makeup for a bride at her wedding but you have no makeup on! Always remember you don't have to be snobby or someone you are not to get ahead. In my experience just being uniquely you is all that's required but please look the part!

**Time out** – Don't be desperate for work but be open to working in a different type of business like a spa or lash lounge for experience until you get what you desire. If you are planning to open a salon please, take your time and get some business courses or a mentor who has a salon first. Be their assistant or protégé for 6 months to a year before investing in your dream. If you booth rent a space in a big salon where others rent space be sure you have enough clientele and don't buy into your landlords sparkling smile. I agree sometimes taking a leap of faith at a high traffic business may work for you but don't be deceived trust me, all that glitters isn't gold. Do your research and play smarter not harder because a good strategy and plan will save you a lot of time and stress later down the line. So, I'm sure your probably thinking how can you stand out from other beauty professionals? Well I'm glad you asked so let's talk about it.

**Professional Documents:** Whether your school has helped you with this or not you must have a beautiful clean resume, cover letter and references. In addition to this beautiful high quality photos in a digital or hard copy portfolio will add to branding and selling yourself to potential employers. Do not use silly font on your resume or symbols. Keep it neat and clean.

**Find A Good Place To Work:** This is the first step to becoming a reputable and distinguished beauty professional. If you work in a well-known salon, you will gain the necessary on-the-job experience that will be invaluable in your quest to carve a niche for yourself. Importantly, make yourself available to clients when other beauticians move on. With that, you will start building a profile that will help launch your brand.

**Promote Yourself:** You must self-promote to gain the desired recognition. If you have been previously timid, this is the time to let go of the habit and get sociable. If you don't promote yourself, it will be difficult for potential clients to know your skills and expertise. You can start by getting friendly with whoever visits the salon and chat up prospective clients. Over time, you will be recognized, and if you do things right, you are good to go.

**Specialize:** Some of us have the capacity to do multiple things well and some of us do not. If you are a Jack-of-all-trades, you may not go far in your career. In the beginning, try to find an area of your profession where you can specialize. You need some ingenuity and good perception to come out with something unique, perhaps a new style or tweaking some old styles to create something fascinating. This will lend credence to your ability and skills. If one or two clients are satisfied with you, you have gotten yourself unpaid advertising agents.

**Be professional and reliable:** Complacency is one of the many challenges of some established beauticians. At some point in their career, they become highly unprofessional and unreliable; shifting schedules to accommodate their conveniences and treating punctuality with disdain. In most cases, such nonchalant attitudes have ended the careers of some of these overconfident beauticians prematurely. Resist the temptation to be complacent. Don't let the little recognition you are getting get into your head. You still have a long way to go. Being professional and reliable will take you to where pride and arrogance can never attain.

**Don't settle for low quality:** As a beginner, the desire to make a living may be challenging. Many beginners addressed that problem by settling for what is below their standards. Then it stuck on them. Getting out of that quandary became a big challenge. If you don't want to be in the same shoes with such individuals, maintain a high standard which we will talk about in a few chapters. If it becomes challenging now to do that, a little patience and endurance will see you through. By then, you will be recognized for your high standards and quality rather settling for less initially and get stuck with it.

However, since the beauty world is highly competitive and challenging, how can you ensure that your clients remain loyal to you so that they will resist the temptation to pledge their allegiance to someone else? I will give you some other useful tips that will always keep your clients rooting for you regardless of the competition, making you the next best thing to happen to the beauty industry.

**Heart to Heart** – Don't forget about your dreams and goals. You are unique and gifted don't let anyone tear down your self-esteem whether peers, business professionals or friends. Yes you got into this to make money but not for money alone, you're an artist now so create, innovate and don't hold back!

After your graduation comes the real challenge of how to distinguish yourself from fellow beauty professionals, let's talk about that.

# CHAPTER 6

## STAY SHARP!

No matter what part of beauty you decide to invest in, you must always learn more about the industry and the business. You will most likely need continuing education classes to renew your licensure in most states. If this is true for you, it's a wonderful way to re-educate yourself each year on the rules and regulations in your area, any changes made by the governing entities. You may also have new areas of interest that you may want to explore, this is a great way to do it and get credit for it. You also want to be aware of CEU scammers, they promise licenses for modalities that don't require a license depending on the state you live in or they teach their own philosophies and in some cases the course has no real use in the industry at all. Be sure the CEU (continuing education unit) provider has an accredited program and the state you reside in has approved the curriculum.

**Tips:**

- Make sure you keep track of your licenses expiration date.

- Renew you CEU'S ahead of time to avoid the "rush" before renewing your license.

- Check you states licensing and regulation website for approved CEU providers list.

- Before your license is due you will get quite a few CEU provider flyers in the mail competing for your business. Shop around for the best price and check to make sure they are approved then read online reviews.

- Make sure you know the difference between CEU's and continuing education courses, not all continuing education will qualify for license renewal.

  Ok so we have talked quite about the process. Let get into how to interact with you peers and customers. Shall we begin?

# CHAPTER 7

## YOUR STANDARD

From the moment a person meets you they can figure out by your body language and appearance what you're about physically. Your sparkling personality can be thrown out the back door to the rats if your first impressions are questionable. Now honestly, there are some employers and people in general that will except you quirky and creative look but depending on how you intend to brand yourself like we discussed earlier, you have to have a standard no matter what it looks like. Whether you're in retail, beauty, sales or the corporate world you must have a standard. Let me help you by painting a picture. So in my family if we see something on the floor that doesn't belong there we pick it up. This expectation is not a standard in some homes so if I visit a friend's house and there is a big ball of tissue on the floor who in the room sees the ball of tissue growing into the size of a snowball minute by minute? Me! They don't care obviously or maybe they don't see it but never the less it's my standard so I will notice it more than others. How about dishes for example wash while cooking dinner or wash after dinner? Which one do you like? I like to cook and clean and others like to watch the dishes pile up! I say all this to say that we all have standards that were taught or discovered. As you explore what your standards are in your life personally and professionally, they will mold other areas of your life like choosing friends, lovers, morals beliefs, integrity and free will. Let's say for example, you witness a really good friend and co-worker stealing products from your job. When you catch them they say to you, " I've put in so much time at this job they owe me, what is a small bottle of shampoo to them they are millionaires". You have two choices at this moment, either give in to the cause and join the 5 finger discount party wagon or use your standards. The bigger picture here is whether friends or not this co-worker is not just stealing from the business but they are also stealing from the team. Come on you mean to tell me you don't want to be a tattle-tale! To have a healthy standard is to make a stand for something so you don't fall for anything. Let's just tell the truth if you don't say anything when your co-worker steals what does it say about you? Not saying anything says everything so now your own standards are on the line and questionable. When you have healthy standards in life your customers, co- workers and even close friends and family can tell. The standards you have in life will build personal and professional relationships or break them.

# CHAPTER 8

## NAVIGATING THE WORKPLACE

Many times in life we often quote the classic biblical principle, treat others how you want to be treated. When it comes to customer service we often expect more than we offer. We want excellent service but we don't give it. When interacting with customers or even the people close to us we must do our best to mirror positivity the best we can, we will fall short but the effort speaks volumes. Not every client will like you no matter how polite you are to them and quite frankly you shouldn't care. You are there to give them an excellent service and experience no matter what. You may not be everyone's favorite person at work and that's ok, just don't acquire the people pleasing syndrome because it will get you nowhere fast. Play nice with rude coworkers and be a team player and help each other but don't enable lazy behavior. There will always be slackers on the job, freeloaders and just plain ol mean people, but don't let them get you down you should not except mess!

I recall a scenario in my career dealing with a co-worker who asked to speak with me in private and I agreed. It was a very busy day at the salon and I had been joking with other co-workers to keep the day in good spirits and fun. We were talking about the heavy workload and how challenging some of the customers were to take care of. One person made fun of a client and we all joked we went about our day and in the last hour of business when the day slowed down form all the hustle and bustle my co-worker asked to speak with me in private. She made mention of the joke we shared earlier about the client and how she was offended because she now felt uncomfortable receiving services from our teammates. She also wondered how we could be so nice to the client and joke behind their backs and then expects the team to not feel awkward receiving services from us. She was going to treat herself to a relaxing spa treatment despite her insecurities about her body. Now she refuses to treat herself at her own spa for fear the co-workers would joke about her. I was dumbfounded, speechless and full of sorrow. Even though the intent wasn't to hurt someone that day I was a part of it and I felt like dirt. She accepted my apology and quit her job and relocated. This woman changed my life because I realized I didn't treat my guests or co-workers the way I wanted be treated directly or indirectly. A harmless joke could be toxic in the workplace along with lack of respect, bad attitudes and selfishness. These behaviors are poison in the workplace and quickly spread like the disease called "drama". The bottom line is you get what you give. You put out good energy you get it back and the same for bad energy believe me you will get it back. In some cases you will put out good energy and still get bad back. Just consider the source it's probably just a sour puss but always do your best to treat others how you want to be treated.

**Replay**

- Remember to treat others how you want to be treated
- Be mindful of your behavior, comments and views in professional environments
- Don't be a Toxic person
- DON'T CREATE DRAMA OR GOSSIP!

# CHAPTER 9

## SERVITUDE

Yes I said it, the customer isn't always right! I mean, no one wants to talk about it. So here's the truth of the matter, I believe customers should always feel comfortable and served. They are paying me for a service and it's my job to make sure their needs are met. However not every customer has good intentions, there are plenty of scammers and freeloaders out there believe me when I tell you I know! I have had a gambit of professional complainers who never had any intention of paying me. I have worked at businesses where the customers have stolen right in front of our faces and challenged us to call the police. I have even had customers try to physically threaten other employees for no apparent reason at all.

Always begin your day asking (in my case asking God) for more capacity to receive pure unconditional love and give pure unconditional love. Without love you cannot give or receive anything let alone serve. And how can you take care of others needs if you are depleted of your own. The airlines always tell you to put your breathing mask before putting on someone else's so that you can help someone else. Remember earlier we talked about *Servant Leadership*, it's simply stating that the best leaders are servants as well. Able to follow and able to lead, able to solve problems and able to let other help solve problems. You get where I'm going here? You will have difficult people to work with in life whether family or friend, co-worker or boss. So study and listen to the people you work with because even if they aren't saying anything they are trying to communicate something and it's your job as the professional to figure it out. Body language is awesome because it just doesn't lie no matter what field you're in! Whether you are in an interview or being interviewed body language can dismiss your chances of hiring someone or getting hired. I recall a woman who always has a snarly twitch in her upper lip every time I spoke with her face to face. I wondered if my breath had a stench or even worst, body odor. Come to find out she hated me and anyone who was in management over her. She had a hard time with leadership and did not last very long at the job because her body language was very tense, angry and sinister. I never had the chance to ask her why she felt this way and I probably wouldn't have received an answer. No matter how nice you are you won't be every ones cup of tea and that's ok as long as you don't allow it to affect you negatively because if you do you will you will take on that persons false view of you and that can lead to poor self-esteem. In other cases, your clients may pull back from you or refuse service from you because of your race this happened to me. They may constantly stare at you or demean you, believe me it will get weird and you will laugh to your self-remembering what you read in this book but now you're prepared!

Some of your clients may be drunk or on drugs the list goes on and on. No matter what you must be ready to help your clients and it may mean calling them a cab because they're tipsy. If your client is coughing get them water and if they are shivering get a blanket or adjust the heater if possible. Need I say more? Its not rocket science just watch them I don't mean stare like a weirdo... just pay attention!

# CHAPTER 10

## THE ART OF RETENTION

My motto is to treat everyone like a VIP (very important person) and I do but, every now and again I get an extraordinary human being in my presence and I extend a little bit more attention to them not because they get preferential treatment but because of their investment in me personally and professionally. I never want you to treat someone differently based on their social economic status, gender or ethnicity. But I do want you to take a good look at the relationships you have personal and professional and take note of how you treat them. Being in the beauty industry for over 15 years you

Can imagine how many services I've done! Out of them all I can recall 7 very special guests that considered me a VIP not just a worker. This type of customer sticks with you through thick in thin, price increases, relocations and leave of absences. It's your core clientele, your stability and livelihood. The core doesn't get better treatment than the other customers, they just get more of you. This is how you build good stable retention. Retention is more than a number it is how you attract and keep your customers. For some it people it is natural and you really just have to show up and be yourself. While others have to learn the art of customer retention and it may take a while. No matter what you must retain customers to succeed and when you really have the ball in your court your core clients will market, advertise and retain future customers for you. So what's my secret you ask? Consistency, microphone drop... it really is that simple!

**Heart to heart:** I have tough days ok especially when I'm cramping ladies, or when I simply love my job but I just don't want to work or talk or smile or look at anyone! Ladies and gentleman its ok to feel this way just take vacations periodically and take a few mental health days.   These clients of yours are buying you...period so give them something worth investing in!

**Tips On Retaining Clients:**

- Be respectful

- No matter how close you get to your clients do not treat them like a BFF (best friend forever)
- Discount services for them when you can afford to
- Invite them to exclusive parties and events
- Send out periodic thank you cards and holiday cards according to their personal observances
- BE CONSISTANT in whatever you provide
- Study the guest and anticipate a need

Let break this down a bit.

**Offer Quality Services:** Nobody will want to re-engage a cosmetologist or massage therapist who turns out to be a time waster. If the services that you offer your customers are of the best quality that can be found anywhere in the world, your customers will always come back to you. A useful trick is to know the latest styles and technologies in the industry and use them for your customers.

**Be Mindful Of Your Grooming and Dressing:** I have previously mentioned this while I was highlighting the qualities that will make you a successful beauty school student. This same quality is needed if you want to retain your customers. Irrespective of your expertise and skills, your grooming is another area you must consider. If you are impeccably dressed, you are advertising yourself, and customers are more likely to consider booking you. Of course, as we mentioned earlier you style and brand need to fit in no matter where your working. Be yourself and be appropriate.

**Have Good Customer Service Skills:** You must have the reputation of being friendly, accommodating, and supportive to your customers. Treat your customers like a king and they will repay that royal treatment with unquestionable loyalty to you.

**Creativity Is A Must:** No customer likes a beautician who refuses to change or grow. If you are not creative, you are practically showing your customers the exit door. However, if you are creative and professional in your approach to your customers and career, you customers will not have any reason to switch their allegiance.

**Make Useful Suggestions:** Your job is to make your customers look and feel great. If you know of a better way to make that happen, don't hesitate to suggest that to your customer. Perhaps you have a new idea of how to apply makeup or perform other procedures, tactfully and professionally sell the idea to your clients.

**Surprise your clients:** Surprise you new clients with a few sample products or randomly choose a client to give a free service to. For example a young man came to visit me for a pedicure and he was hungry, I asked what do you like he said a burger fries and beer but I'll wait until I get home. So I told him I was going to grab something for his treatment but really I ordered his food and I paid for it. He gave me a large tip which I didn't expect but he was surprised and felt special. Another quick example is an empathetic surprise for clients who are going through a divorce, lost a job or loved one. Sometimes a complimentary hand or scalp massage, flowers or a free service helps in times of distress. Who wouldn't want to hear your massage is on me or your haircut is on the house. This is easy when its you own business but most employers are pretty open to these things as long as they have a heads up.

We've had extensive discussion on what it takes to be a good industry professional, from finding the best school to retaining your clients. The useful tips mentioned during the course of the discussion will guide you from school and throughout your career. Did I just mention career? You haven't thought of that? Now that I have mentioned it, what are the possible job opportunities that are available to you? I will discuss some of them.

# CHAPTER 11

## NO LIMITS

### CAREER OPPORTUNITIES IN COSMETOLOGY

There are no limits to the job opportunities that are available to you so create! Create a job for yourself no one has done before. Here a just a few examples of what's available to you:

**Medical Esthetician:** Although no state has an actual medical license solely for this modality. Some medical doctors under their supervision will train you on some medical procedures. If you are a nurse or medical assistant , becoming an esthetician will get you into to doctors offices very quickly and with higher pay than most new graduates.

**Cosmetology Instructor:** This is an opportunity to share the knowledge you have acquired over time with new students, teach skills and sanitation procedures required by your local state .

**Fashion Show Stylist:** There are dozens of fashion shows all over the world. You will have the opportunity to showcase your talent at these fashion shows.

**Beauty Magazine Editor:** As a professional, your expertise will be instrumental to churning out beauty articles that can change the fashion world.

**Cosmetology School Owner:** Imagine having your own beauty school! That will be a great experience you won't like to trade for anything.

**Education and Training:** One of my personal favorites because in this career path you may travel to teach staff members or represent a retail brand.

This is an inexhaustible list not to mention you may come up with an even better path that's unique and in high demand so go for it!

There are tons of other job opportunities that you may try to launch a career in.

**Freelance:** Not really into big salon/spas with lots of employees? Maybe a freelancing your services is better for you. Just make sure you get lots of training in all the modalities you want to offer so that you will be highly recommended with lots of booked gigs.

There is so much to do, like microblading, eye lash extensions, makeup, nail art and more! Just follow your states guidelines and get the proper training as a licensed professional. Safety, sanitation and customer service remember! Create contracts for your clients and set deposits for your services so that your clients are sure they have retained you for an event.

# Conclusion

I hope you have now found some useful tips that will help you overcome your fears and launch yourself to a successful career in the beauty world.

Rome was not built in a day; a successful career in any field does not happen over night it happens on purpose. If you are reading this book its book its because your have purpose and a call on your life that is higher than you can even imagine. I want to help you unlock that gift with wisdom and preparation. Therefore, take some of these useful tips and consider them carefully to determine whether you are cut out for a career in this multi-billion dollar industry.

If you've discovered that your future lies in this profession, read this book again from the beginning and use it as a guide to help you make the right decision at every stage of your career.

With diligence and determination, you will launch a career that will guarantee you financial freedom and recognition. My hope is that you will not make the same mistakes so many pros have made in the past. I pretty sure you will have bumps in the road    to success but with this guide I know you will succeed in places you couldn't even imagine!

# ABOUT THE AUTHOR

Amber Rowe is an author, speaker, beauty coach and licensed nail technician with over 15 years of experience in the beauty industry.
Amber's passion for education began when she realized a decline in the practice and methods of new and licensed beauty professionals in our country.
Her mission is to cultivate  students, eradicate unprofessionalism and preserve the future of the beauty industry one student at a time.
Amber currently resides in Austin, Texas where she enjoys life with her husband and 2 daughters. Her powerful legacy continues through the many students she trains to this day.